50 JUICING RECIPES

For Weight Loss and Healthy Living

EMMA GREEN

Book

6

CONTENTS

FOREWORD

"I love everything about Emma's connection to weight loss and health."

Hi, my name is Nat Lee, and I've spent most of my life looking pretty good and feeling great. That was up until I started eating on the run and allowing my busy life as a mom to take hold of me. While working too.

In truth, I knew I should eat great food, but time constraints and "motherly craziness" got the better of me. I made sure my son ate well. But I didn't, which was silly, really. Parenting is one of those things that just takes over your life, I suppose. So, anyway, I kinda ate loads of stuff I shouldn't, and drank sodas and milkshakes an awful lot. Chocolate and takeout became my best friend, and I became overweight, by anyone's standards. No one really told me I looked bad, I mean, most people aren't that obvious. But when I was diagnosed with a severe illness and bedridden for four years, it became time to do something to help my recovery. I made the change as soon as I could.

Since reading Emma's books, I've lost 18.5 kg (which is 40 amazing pounds). And I've managed to keep it off by following her wonderful advice, and by using her awesome, easy-to-do recipes. I live relatively simply, but her guide to nutrition and her tips and tricks have helped me a bucket load. Thank you Emma, you've literally changed my life!

INTRODUCTION

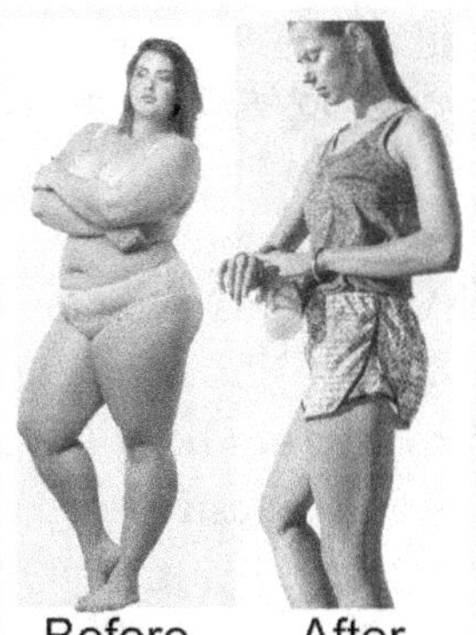

Hi! And thank you so much for joining me here in my book! My name is Emma Green, and I am so excited to share with you my most favorite recipe ideas for juicing, for the purposes of healthy living and weight loss, combined.

Growing up, I learned to love my southern lifestyle. It was cheaper to eat badly than it was to get fresh produce at the time. We didn't have heaps of money and we got by as best we could. So, my mom got what was cheap when we ventured to the local store. The food was inexpensive, and my mother made us the best meals, despite us living below the poverty line. When you're poor, you tend to eat more calorie-dense foods because they're actually cheaper than fruits and vegetables, and that's just how it was for us. I don't blame Mom for spoiling me, because, in reality, she didn't know any better. The only difference nowadays, is that we are noticing the effects that modern day (westernized) diets have on the body as a whole.

Please know, if you haven't already read my title, "How I Lost 100 Pounds! My Personal Weight Loss Strategies for Optimum Happiness," make sure you get your FREE copy today. Inside you'll learn exactly how I lost my weight, and the benefits of knowing the must-do nutrition, and other amazing secrets including myths, water weight, cellulite prevention and removal, the only exercise you really need, the ancient and easy technique to help slim you quickly, how to balance meals, and much, much more! I hope you love it. It's my very special gift to you!

The importance of healthy living is paramount to all of us, and ultimately so that we can live long, illness-free lives. And to achieve that goal, we must be willing to give our body the sustenance it needs on a nutrient-based level, and so that it can sustain itself for the long term.

In the case of weight loss, I personally believe that it's a detrimental part of health to be the best, most awesome version of you – for your amazing journey into feeling good, and so that the body can be working smarter (not harder) to sustain itself and remain illness free. Like a plant, if you give it exactly the right mix of nutrients, it will grow; healthily, beautifully and without wilting or dying. If we think of our own body like a plant, we can understand (from a simplistic viewpoint) that we need to do the same. And if we know what it needs, then "presto" we just have to feed it!

I want you to know that I am coming from a place of actually doing this myself. I tried loads of things to get the body I wanted over the years; for health and weight loss achievement, together. I have utilized juicing as a major part of my ongoing health regime, and I now (definitely) look and feel amazing, especially compared to how I used to! So, let's keep going, I want to talk with you about a few things before we get started. Then you can have some fun with my all-time favorite recipe ideas for juicing! Thanks again for stopping by. I truly wish you every success in your health and wellness journey. And - if you're trying to lose weight, you've definitely come to the right place!

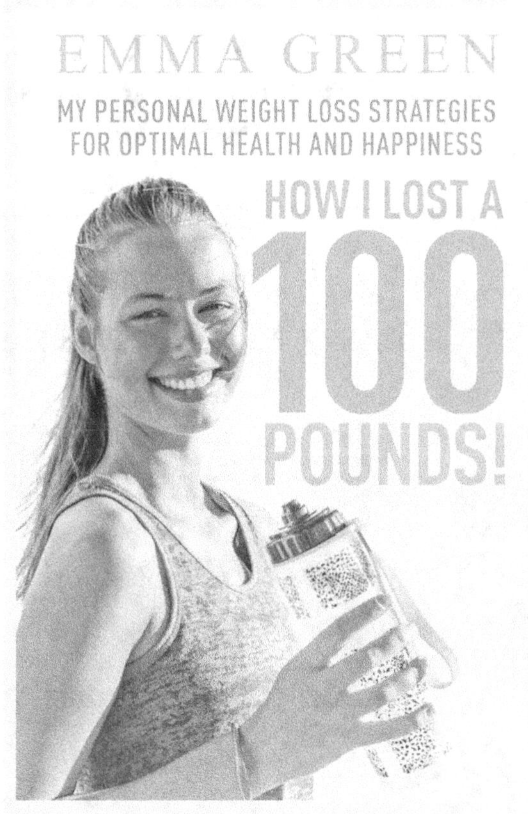

Btw check out "How i lost a 100 pounds" if you haven't already, its got loads of value and its completely FREE :)

FREE GIFTS!

Here are 3 bonus books I want to gift you for coming and reading this title! Sign up to my newsletter and you will receive:

Weight Loss Myths - 9 myths that you are mostly likely doing right now that are totally pointless and are a waste of time toward your weight loss goals.

How to Lose Weight Fast – A 10 day plan I personally put together to make that weight literally melt before your eyes (it worked for me!)

And... Weight Loss Secrets - Secrets the main stream media and health industry never talk about because (let's be honest) things that work don't make them money!

Click here to sign up! or for paperback versions grab it through the ebook completely FREE!

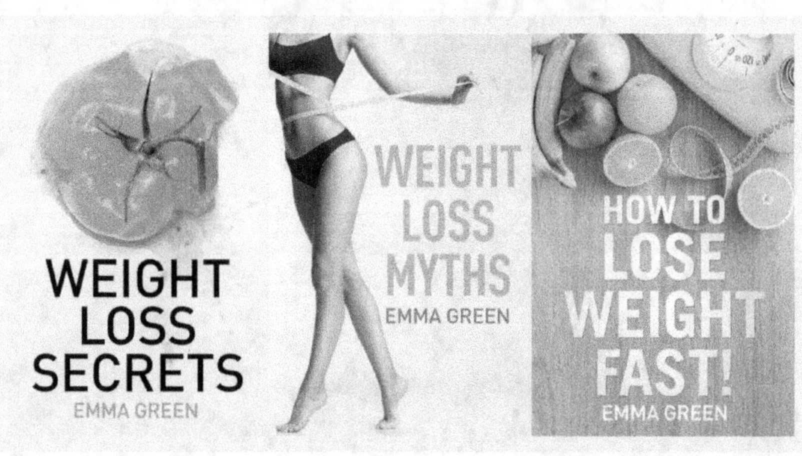

THE HEALTH ISSUES FROM A CONVENTIONAL US-BASED DIET

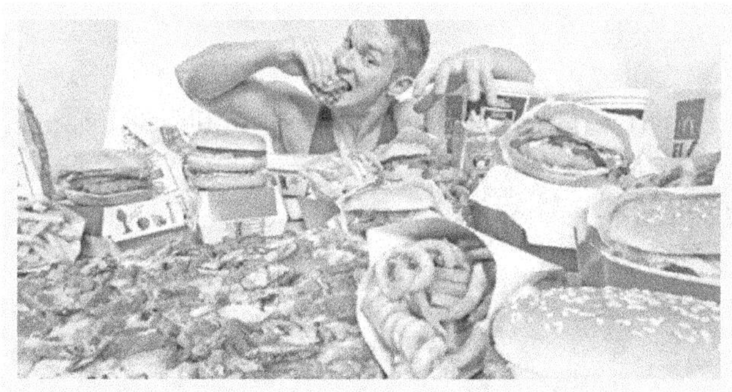

Statistically speaking, the health issues climbing in the US are at an alarmingly high rate. Many statistics show us that illnesses like heart disease, cancer, diabetes (type 1 and 2), are on the rise, and phenomenally so. There are other illnesses that have been linked to poor diet and lifestyle factors, too. They include: ADHD, stroke, dementia, Alzheimer's disease, Parkinson's disease, and many, many more.

Unfortunate Statistics:

- Unhealthy diets contribute to 678,000 deaths per year in the US
- Obesity rates have doubled in the US for adults in the past 30 years
- Obesity rates have tripled in the US for children in the past 30 years
- Obesity rates have quadrupled in the US for adolescents in the past 30 years
- Recent reports project that half of all adults will be obese by the year 2030, and that's just in the US alone
- Poor eating habits and lack of physical activity are the top 2 reasons contributing to weight and obesity, globally

Changing the Way That We Live:

A healthy diet that gives us fuel or energy should always made up of a good proportion of fruits and vegetables (80% of daily intake is suggested). The rest should be grains, meat, fish, and variations like eggs, and minimal dairy, if any.

As kids, we were taught good eating habits at school, and hopefully by our parents, too. Unfortunately, nowadays, the trend is about the hype and pleasure of the ease of fast food; not nutritional food, as a necessity. As a result, we have seen the fast food industry blow out, to one that is now booming, ridiculously. And also, it's because "we," as a collective, are far too busy to put our health first, so "we" suffer and have health issues as a result. Our lack of focus is due to time spent at jobs, looking after kids, being responsible for a family, spending time with friends, and other areas of our lives that take up copious amounts of our time.

If we took just an hour per day to make sure we were eating right, our whole world would change, definitively so! Yes, it's true, and I know because I did it myself! I really can tell you - that you can definitely feel better, look better, and be functioning at your greatest capacity, with weight loss added as the real bonus to great health. Yes!! Weight loss is a viable and very-achievable goal here!

THE BENEFITS OF JUICING FOR WEIGHT LOSS

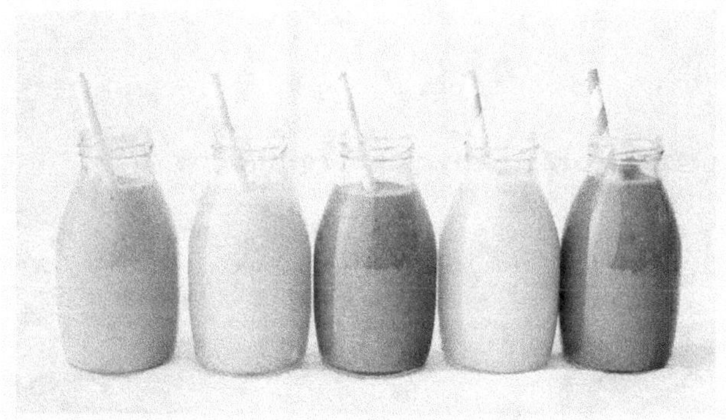

My aunt and my mom were talking loudly in the living room and discussing my uncle Frank's high blood sugar level. He received the news after his doctor ran some tests. I was bringing the tea in and I wondered whether he might be able to lower it with juicing. I knew it had loads of benefits, other than just weight loss.

I explained the benefits of juicing to my aunt Clara. She immediately began asking me how she could do it. So, after we finished our tea, we went into the kitchen and I showed her some of my favorite recipes. I let her take some home for my uncle. Turns out he absolutely loved them.

It took one month, but the doctor was astonished when the levels came back nearly normal. He said, "Whatever you're doing keep doing it!" And sent him home with a smile on his face. He rang me that night to thank me. Aunt Clara was over the moon!

This is one of my favorite stories, because my family means everything to me. And if you can help them through knowledge sharing, then it's awesome and has wonderful benefits down the line. Because now he'll tell some more people, and then they will, too... and on and on it goes. A cycle of extraordinary good health for everyone! Well, that's the plan.

The Importance of Cruciferous Vegetables:

Cruciferous vegetables can be defined as: vegetables in the Brassicaceae family. Broccoli, cabbage, bok choy, and watercress are examples.

Thankfully, we are not helpless in our exposure to hormone-disrupting chemicals. The foods of the twenty-first century have been made up of many hormone-disrupting chemicals, unfortunately. And a good rule of thumb is; if it comes in a packet and has additives of any kind, there's a good chance it's on the "no-go" list. So, blessedly, this is where the cruciferous vegetables list comes in. The big terms mentioned here are substances: DIM (diindolylmethane) and I3C (indole-3-carbinol). All cruciferous vegetables are rich sources of these wonderful phytonutrients. So, let's see...

DIM (diindolylmethane) and I3C (indole-3-carbinol) can contribute to:

- Improving Metabolism
- Detoxification
- Hormonal Balance Control
- Blood Sugar Level Control
- Reducing Inflammation in the Body
- Body Fat Reduction

Ultimately, these can mean REAL weight loss! Cruciferous vegetables also have their role in helping your body to keep cancer away. Your mommy was absolutely right when she urged you to eat your broccoli!

Cruciferous Vegetables List:

- Cauliflower (white or purple)
- Broccoli (green or purple)
- Brussels Sprouts
- Kale (green or purple)
- Bok Choy
- Cabbage (green, red or purple)
- Watercress
- Radish
- Broccoli sprouts
- Arugula (rocket)
- Kohlrabi (white or purple)
- Turnip
- Daikon

JUICING RECIPES ARE AWESOME FOR WEIGHT LOSS AND A HEALTHY DIGESTIVE TRACT:

One day when I was preparing to juice, my friend Julianne came over. She looked at me as I chopped up my fruit and vegetables. She asked me what I was making, and could she have the recipe for it. When I told her about juicing, and the addition of great stuff like chia seeds and superfoods, she gave me a big smile. "Em, do you reckon my boys might drink it? Gosh, I have been trying, and failing, to give them vegetables. I feel like a terrible mother, sometimes."

I smiled at her. "Oh absolutely, yes! I think they'll definitely love them."

Julianne stayed for over an hour that day, and I showed her how easy it was to do. She went to the store on her way home and bought a good quality juicer. Her boys love drinking them now, and they have even showed their friends how to do it, too. She was stunned when they asked if they could make them after school with their friends.

She rang me the next week and asked me for more recipes. "I need more, the boys say. And ones with their favorite fruits!" This prompted me to write this title. Now, I can share my recipes with everyone. They're totally kid-friendly! I know you'll love them too!

The whole cruciferous family are spectacularly known for their soothing and healing effects on the digestive system. A healthy digestive tract is of crucial importance when it comes to your absorption of vital nutrients listed in their scientific terms, as we saw earlier. And so… just by using awesome juicing recipes that include cruciferous veggies, you will actually improve the nutrient absorption capacity, and the ease (in terms of functionality) for your entire body as a whole.

In a sense, your juicer breaks down the added produce, so that your body can assimilate the nutrients with functional ease.

Tip: You can further increase the uptake of the nutrients by adding a portioned amount of healthy fat when ingesting your juice. This can be done in a number of ways; sprinkle some freshly ground flax or pumpkin seeds into the juice, as an example. Or, you could add some coconut, a slice of avocado, or an addition of peanut butter on a celery stalk.

Fruit and Vegetables Are Awesome:

Fruit and vegetables are full of phytonutrients, vitamins, minerals and antioxidants that build your natural immunity. Amazingly, they support your eyes, bones, hormone balance, heart, metabolism, digestion and cell health.

Weight Loss Awesomeness:

If you have been on a lot of diets and eating improperly for a long time, utilizing juicing recipes are an effective way to nudge your body into shedding fat and also to help in keeping it off, long term. When you are carrying more weight around, then your fat cells become toxic. Juicing can amazingly help you clean your entire system. You need to nourish your cells back to health and accelerate the fat loss through nutrient supplementation.

The ultra-amazing thing is, that you will (in essence) be totally altering your body's biochemistry to a more alkaline state. An alkaline state (a PH level achievement around 7.4 internally) allows for homeostasis (a perfect, internal, cellular harmony) and it also shields disease and illness, too. It's known to knock out cancer (see Dr. Otto Warburg for more on that — you will love reading his discoveries). It's kind of like magic, really. Some health promoters and scientists have also come to believe that juicing regularly is the way to increase your insulin sensitivity and reverse type 2 diabetes - and many other illnesses that are not reversed with western medicine. Those topics are for another book, or books.

Important Facts:

- When you have fat, your body needs to become alkaline (not acidic) and you need to recalibrate.
- Enzymes are the spark for the thousands of biochemical reactions in the body; the substances that act as catalysts that control all the life processes.
- Fruit and vegetables are involved in all bodily functions. Raw, fresh fruit and vegetable juices are full of living enzymes. They are the elixir of life!

Enzymes:

There are 2 types of enzymes; digestive and metabolic. It's the metabolic enzymes that are responsible for detoxification processes and energy production in the body. When you are overweight, it's the metabolic processes that are impaired. The best way to rejuvenate your health and lose weight is by juicing plenty of fruits and vegetables every single day.

Dietary Tips to Aid with Juicing for Weight Loss:

You must remove all processed sugars from your diet; this includes the high-glycemic foods (food groups metabolized quickly through digestion and absorption), high-density carbohydrates, or the starch-filled foods, as a rule of definite incorporation.

Concentrate on removing breads, chocolates, crackers, potato chips, soda, pancakes, cakes, and fast food meals that are high in carbs or sugars to aid your diet.

Juicing recipes for weight loss are meant to replace heavy meals once a day. You can drink your favorite juice before your evening meal and make that meal a low-glycemic snack, rather than a complete meal.

Raw juices are highly therapeutic and will improve the quality of your diet! If you have a lot of fat to lose there is no better way to ensure your health, energy, and the synergy of awesome metabolic functioning than to utilize juicing, as a definitive way of life. It has changed mine, thankfully; and unbelievably so! Now, I get to share my most awesome recipes with you!

Chapter One

50 MOST AWESOME JUICING RECIPES

RECIPE #1: BEAUTIFUL BEETS PLUS

Ingredient List:

- 180g of beetroot (1 beet)
- 50g or two leaves of cabbage (red)
- 190g (3 medium) carrots
- 50g (1/2 a fruit) lemon
- 140g (1 whole) orange
- 230g (1/4 a fruit) pineapple
- 60g (1 handful) spinach

Directions:

When ready, simply process all the ingredients together in your favorite blender. You can shake it up or stir it up, then serve and enjoy.

Helpful Tips: Smooth It Out

To create a smoother consistency, you can add an inch or two of water.

This will create a less dense mixture, and will make your juice easier to ingest. I always add any leaves last.

Amazing Facts: Pineapples

Pineapples are helpful to create an ease in body digestion as well as helping to rid the body of inflammation, therefore creating a bounty of vitamin C to your juice. Vitamin C is great to ward off colds and flu and helps the immune system to boost itself vitally.

Chapter Two

RECIPE #2: APPLE MAID

Ingredient List:

- 730g (4 medium) apples
- 200g (3 stalks) of celery
- 70g (2 leaves) of kale
- 60g (1 whole lemon – peeled)
- 130g (4 cups) of spinach

Directions:

Start by chopping your apples, celery, and the lemon into slices or bigger pieces. Put these items into your blender, then add kale and celery, and blitz it all up, until smooth. Shake it up and enjoy.

Helpful Tips: Leave the Peel On

Leaving the skin on the well-washed apples will enable your body to ingest the goodness from the part of the fruit that is often tossed aside. You can do this with the lemon, too.

Amazing Facts: Awesome Apples

Apples have amazing nutrients inside of them. Jam packed, full of vitamin A, vitamin C, magnesium, and protein. Your body utilizes all of these vitamins and minerals to function properly and sufficiently. We definitely love apples!

Chapter Three

RECIPE #3: GREEN TWIST SURPRISE

Ingredient List:

- 370g (2 medium) apples
- 80g (2 stalks) of celery
- 300g (1 whole) cucumber
- 180g (5 leaves) of kale
- 50g (1/2 fruit) lemon
- 270g (2 whole) oranges
- 40g (1 handful) of parsley

Directions:

Chop the parsley and kale together, then dice the apple, cucumber, celery, lemon, and oranges into bigger, bulkier chunks. Put all ingredients into a blender and blitz until smooth. Stir, and pour into a glass, then enjoy.

Helpful Tips: Love Yourself First

Taking care of you is important. Your health relies on it, actually! Get enough rest and make sure you stay as stress-free as possible. Weight loss can be achieved when you love yourself first!

Amazing Facts: The Beauty of Oranges

There are only 47 calories per 100 grams in every orange. Packed full of vitamins and minerals like: vitamin A, calcium, vitamin C, magnesium, and vitamin B-6. Wow! All that goodness in just one ingredient!

Chapter Four

RECIPE #4: COOLIO AWESOME

Ingredient List:

- 60g (2 cups) of spinach
- 60g (1 whole) lemon
- 140g (4 leaves) of kale
- 300g (1 whole) cucumber
- 370g (2 medium) apples

Directions:

Just dice your apples and cucumber into manageable, bigger-sized chunks and put them into your juicer. Add other ingredients. Blitz the full entourage until smooth, and serve with loads of ice.

Helpful Tips: Using Ice to Accentuate

Crushed ice works nicely and makes an icy-styled drink which can be great for kids too. It's awesome in the summertime!

Amazing Facts: Chillin' with Cucumbers

Cucumber is highly beneficial for the body. They contain vitamin K and molybdenum. Important for nail health, they also contain the promotion mineral called silica. Other minerals include: copper, potassium, manganese, magnesium, and biotin. Vitamins C and B1 are also inside them. Wow, cucumbers are amazing!

Chapter Five

RECIPE #5: COOL AS A CUCUMBER

Ingredient List:

- 550g (3 whole) apples
- 200g (3 stalks) of celery
- 150g (1/2 vegetable) cucumber
- 10g (1/2 thumb) of ginger root
- 140g (4 leaves) of kale
- 60g (1 whole) lemon
- 180g (1 whole large) orange - peeled

Directions:

Dice celery, cucumber, lemon, apples, and ginger root into bigger chunks. Add the kale, and blitz the full mixture until smooth. Serve raw and cold.

Helpful Tips: Plan Ahead

Plan ahead: the week, the month, and even the year. Being organized can help you to achieve goals for weight loss and in other areas of your life too!

Amazing Facts: Lovely Lemons

Lemons contain vital nutrients. They are rich in vitamin C, which is an important ingredient to help protect the body against immune deficiencies. Lemons also contain pectin fiber which is super-beneficial for colon health. Gotta love that!

Chapter Six

RECIPE #6: FRUIT AND VEGETABLE CREATION

Ingredient List:

- 90g (3 cups) of spinach
- 130g (2 stalks) of celery
- 460g (8 medium) carrots
- 180g (1 whole) beet
- 180g (1 medium) apple

Directions:

Simply chop all the ingredients into smaller-sized chunks and add them to your juicer. Blitz until smooth and serve cold.

Helpful Tips: Overnight's A Charm

You can leave this juice overnight and drink as a refreshing morning pick-me-up. The flavors and the nutrients will aid your body all day long.

Amazing Facts: Super-Duper Celery

Celery is awesome! Celery contains antioxidants and beneficial enzymes as well. They also contain loads of vitamins and minerals like vitamin K, vitamin C, potassium, folate, and vitamin B6. How does it all fit in there? Amazing, right?

Chapter Seven

RECIPE #7: BEET TREAT

Ingredient List:

- 20g (1/2 thumb) of ginger root
- 150g (1/2 vegetable) cucumber
- 200g (3 stalks) of celery
- 250g (4 medium) carrots
- 180 (1 whole) beet
- 370g (2 medium) apples

Directions:

Just chop all the ingredients into medium chunks and pour them into your juicer. Blitz until smooth, stir, and enjoy.

Helpful Tips: What Do You Need?

Make a list of your juicing week requirements the week beforehand. Then you can put the grocery list with your other needs, and be ready for the week ahead.

Amazing Facts: Terrific Beets

Beets contain amazing nutrients. They can reduce inflammation, support your heart and protect your digestive, brain, and eye health, too! Wow, that's super-awesome!

Amazing Facts: Terrific Beets

Chapter Eight

RECIPE #8: ROOTS AND BEETS

Ingredient List:

- 180g (1 whole) beetroot
- 610g (10 medium) carrots
- 130g (1 full) sweet potato

Directions:

Add the ingredients: Beetroot, followed by the diced sweet potato, followed by the diced carrots. Once the mixture is smooth and silky, pour into a short glass and enjoy.

Helpful Tips: Carrot Peel

Leaving the peel on the carrots is beneficial. Carrot peel that's well-washed contains phytonutrients. These are found in the skin and just underneath the surface, too.

Amazing Facts: Phytonutrients Rock

The definition of a phytonutrient is: a certain plant that has the capacity to be beneficial to health and help in the prevention of various diseases.

Chapter Nine

RECIPE #9: GOOD VIBES

Ingredient List:

- 180g (1 full) beetroot
- 130g (2 stalks) of celery
- 90g (3 cups) of spinach
- 30g (1 teaspoon) of spirulina - dried

Directions:

Chop the celery, beetroot, and spinach. Add to juicer. Add the spirulina and blitz until smooth. Drink when ready.

Helpful Tips: Add A Snack

Juicing is awesome because you can add a snack to your juice for breakfast and lunch each day. The calories are low and weight loss is promoted. You can still have a main meal at night, but add a juice, of course!

Amazing Facts: Vitamin A is Marvelous

Vitamins allow the body to function better. Vitamin A plays a pivotal role in the maintenance of vision, neurological functioning, healthy skin promotion, reducing inflammation, and fighting free radical damage.

Chapter Ten

RECIPE #10: ORANGE AND RED TASTY

Ingredient List:

- 180g (1 whole) beetroot
- 130g (2 medium) carrots
- 260g (2 whole) oranges

Directions:

Chop all ingredients and add them to your juice, together. Blend until smooth then serve cold. Add any garnish you like.

Helpful Tips: You Can Do Anything

The brain is very powerful. Did you know that you can do anything you want, especially when you believe it's possible? Yes, you definitely can. And I am here cheering you on, 100%, and all the way. Positivity helps a real-lot.

Amazing Facts: Marvelous Magnesium

Magnesium: known as the anti-stress mineral, it converts blood sugar to energy. Calcium: initiates DNA synthesis and helps bone health maintenance.

Chapter Eleven

RECIPE #11: TANGY TANGO SMOOTHIE

Ingredient List:

- 60g (2 cups) of spinach
- 30g (1/2 fruit) lime
- 15g (1 whole) jalapeno
- 30g (2 stalks) of celery
- 360g (5 large) carrots
- 180g (1 whole) beetroot

Directions:

Chop the carrots, celery, and beetroot. Now add them to your juicer with the whole jalapeno, ginger root, peeled lime, and the finally, the spinach. Blitz the mixture until smooth and then enjoy. You can de-seed the jalapeno before you add it, if you want to lessen the spicy flavor.

Helpful Tips: Keep It or Lose It

Maintain the hotness or get rid of the jalapeno. It's up to you. Maybe just use it as a garnish if you don't want to drink it in your juice.

Amazing Facts: Jovial Jalapenos

Jalapenos are beneficial to the body because they literally burn calories and fat. The heat created helps you to sweat out the excess water weight.

Chapter Twelve

RECIPE #12: SWEET N' NICE SURPRISE

Ingredient List:

- 370g (2 medium) apples
- 180g (1 whole) beetroot
- 70g (1 large) carrot
- 130g (1 whole) orange
- 130g (1 whole) sweet potato

Directions:

Peel the orange and the carrot, and chop them. Dice the other ingredients into chunks. Add the full mixture to your juicer and blend until smooth and silky. Drink when ready.

Helpful Tips: The Peel is Beneficial

Leaving the peel on the apples, sweet potatoes and carrots is beneficial. Lots of nutrients can be ingested in the peel. Just make sure they are well-washed first. Unreal peel!

Amazing Facts: Low GI Sweet Potato

Sweet potatoes are great. They are low GI which allows the energy to be given to your body over a longer period of time. That's a great way to keep blood sugar levels balanced.

Chapter Thirteen

RECIPE #13: GINGER ROOT CRAZY

Ingredient List:

- 220g (1 large) apple
- 100g (3 leaves) of beet greens
- 180g (1 whole) beetroot
- 250g (4 medium) carrots
- 70g (1 stalk) of celery
- 10g (1/2 a thumb) of ginger root

Directions:

Slice the ginger root into smallish sections, do this along with the celery and beet greens. Add those ingredients to your juicer. Now dice your apple, carrots, and then the beetroot. Blitz together. Leave overnight and enjoy the very next morning.

Helpful Tips: Take It with You

Just because you are headed to work, that doesn't mean that you can't take your juice with you. Just add a cooler pack and "Voila!" you can be healthy anywhere at all. Woo hoo!

Amazing Facts: Gorgeous Ginger Root

Ginger root is beneficial to the body because it can do amazing things. It has the ability to reduce nausea, be used as motion sickness cure, and it can also aid in reducing muscle pain and soreness. Who knew?

Chapter Fourteen

RECIPE #14: RASPBERRY DELICIOUS

Ingredient List:

- 180g (1 whole) beetroot
- 40g (1/2 fruit) lemon
- 540g (3 medium) pears
- 120g (1 cup) raspberries

Directions:

Peel your lemon. You need to leave the skin on your pears. Chop up the lemon, beetroot and pears into cube-sized pieces. Just place the entire mix into your juicer. Blitz until silky, then shake and serve.

Helpful Tips: Add Liquid

Sometimes adding an inch or two of water is beneficial to aid in a smoother consistency, and for easier ingestion. Use rainwater or clean water. Not tap water, because it has loads of chemicals.

Amazing Facts: Wonderful Water

Water makes up between 50-65% of the human body. This is dependent upon the size and leanness of an individual's tissue. Fatty tissue contains less water than lean tissue.

Chapter Fifteen

RECIPE #15: SMOOTH BLEND OF YUMMY

Ingredient List:

- 190g (1 medium) apple
- 180g (1 whole) beetroot
- 740g (12 medium) carrots
- 50g (1/2 fruit) lemon
- 270g (2 whole) oranges - peeled

Directions:

Peel orange, lemon, carrots, beetroot, and apple into larger-sized chunks. Place into your juicer, and let it blend until the mix is smooth. Serve icy cold with ice cubes if you want to.

Helpful Tips: A Powerful Juicer Is Paramount

Make sure you have a powerful juicer that's cleaned well and maintained properly. If not cleaned with hot water, bacteria can grow on its surface. It's important that health is always maintained where food is concerned.

Amazing Facts: Juicing Is Easy and Great for Health

Juicing can aid weight loss and health unbelievably when done properly. The ingredients used are paramount to the success. Fending off illness and longevity can also be achieved. Feeling amazing is the added bonus.

Chapter Sixteen

RECIPE #16: TOMMY TOMATO

Ingredient List:

- 1 tomato
- 1 cucumber
- large handful cilantro
- 3 small zucchinis
- 2 celery sticks

Directions:

Chop vegetables. Add a cup of water if you have a blender because the fiber will be left in the mix. Blend until silky, and enjoy.

Helpful Tips: Nutrient Availability

Leave the skins on to provide even more nutrient availability. When you use the peel, you get more nutrient value. And you won't even know if it's well-blitzed.

Amazing Facts: Lovin' the Tomatoes

Tomatoes are beneficial for health because they aid in: prevention of cancer, skin maintenance, bone health, providing essential antioxidants, and are great for your heart. Wow!

Chapter Seventeen

RECIPE #17: LEMON-GINGER TINGLE

Ingredient List:

- 1 bunch of cilantro
- half head of bok choy
- 1 apple
- squeeze of fresh lemon
- 1/4 teaspoon grated ginger

Directions:

Chop vegetables. Add a cup of water if you have a blender because the fiber will be left in the mix. Blend until silky, and enjoy.

Helpful Tips: Let the Kids Try

We all know how hard it is to keep our kids healthy, so let them help you and experiment with them in the kitchen. If we can get the next generation on board with healthy eating, we can help change the current trending statistics on a wider health scale.

Amazing Facts: Yummy Bok Choy

Bok choy is awesome for health. It aids in: bone health, heart health, inflammation, immunity, and skin health. Wow, loads of benefits there!

RECIPE #18: ITALIAN STALLION

Ingredient List:

- 1 bunch spinach
- 1 handful Italian parsley
- 1 cucumber
- 1 tomato

Directions:

Chop vegetables. Add a cup of water if you have a blender because the fiber will be left in the mix. Blend until silky, and enjoy.

Helpful Tips: Grow It

Growing parsley can be done easily. You don't need a big space or area and you can easily place it in a pot. Add it to everything. Parsley is a fundamental herb for human consumption.

Amazing Facts: Beneficial Parsley

Parsley has great benefits to health. This herb is amazing for strengthening immunity, and works on different aspects of the immune system. Parsley contains: vitamin C, vitamin A, vitamin K, folate, and niacin. A truly magnificent herb!

Chapter Nineteen

RECIPE #19: SIMPLE JUICE

Ingredient List:

- 1 bunch kale
- 3 celery sticks
- 1 apple

Directions:

Chop vegetables. Add a cup of water if you have a blender because the fiber will be left in the mix. Blend until silky, and enjoy.

Helpful Tips: Simple and Effective

Sometimes simple recipes are the most beneficial. You can add as many herbs and/or spices as you wish. Jalapenos are great for aiding weight loss if you can handle their spicy heat. Even if you just add a touch to your recipe, that's awesome!

Amazing Facts: Bountiful Kale

Kale is low in calories, high in fiber and has no fat content at all! It aids the digestive system and helps with bowel movements, too. It's super-duper great for health.

Chapter Twenty

RECIPE #20: GREEN AND ORANGE SPRITZ

Ingredient List:

- 3 carrots
- 1 bunch of spinach
- 1 apple

Directions:

Chop vegetables. Add a cup of water if you have a blender because the fiber will be left in the mix. Blend until silky, and enjoy.

Helpful Tips: Add Honey

If you want to sweeten a juice, you can add a tablespoon of honey. Organic is great because it's the most beneficial for health. In fact, organic anything is always recommended so you can be free of harmful chemicals and/or additives.

Amazing Facts: Carotene Helps

Carotene is the red or orange pigmentation found in carrots and other plants too. It helps the body by aiding as an antioxidant which essentially protects the cells against damage.

Chapter Twenty-One

RECIPE #21: THE SPINACH, CELERY AND TOMATO

Ingredient List:

- 1 - 2 tomatoes
- 1 bunch spinach
- 2 celery sticks

Directions:

Chop vegetables. Add a cup of water if you have a blender because the fiber will be left in the mix. Blend until silky, and enjoy.

Helpful Tips: Positivity Is Beneficial

Stay positive during your weight loss journey. It will be hard some days, but you are so worth it! Listen to music while you work out, or watch a movie when you get time. Spoil yourself rotten.

Amazing Facts: Cherry Tomatoes

Baby tomatoes are full of fiber, vitamin C, and a good dose of other awesome vitamins and minerals. They help the eyes to function and are also have anti-carcinogen properties. They help in weight loss promotion too.

Chapter Twenty-Two

RECIPE #22: ZUMBA FRESH

Ingredient List:

- 3 zucchinis
- 2 celery sticks
- 1 cucumber
- 1 apple

Directions:

Chop vegetables. Add a cup of water if you have a blender because the fiber will be left in the mix. Blend until silky, and enjoy.

Helpful Tips: Meditation is Super

Staying stress free is super-important. Using meditation on a regular basis is great for the mind and the body. It helps to calm and soothe the individual, especially when done regularly.

Amazing Facts: Calcium for Health

Calcium is essential for the body to build and maintain strong and healthy bones. The heart, muscles and nerves all need calcium to function well.

Chapter Twenty-Three

RECIPE #23: MANGO SWIRL BONANZA

Ingredient List:

- 1 cup of unsweetened hemp milk or almond milk
- squeeze of lemon juice
- 2 fresh mangoes
- 1 dried mango
- 1 tablespoon of almond butter
- a sprinkle of flaxseeds
- half a teaspoon of Maca powder
- half a teaspoon of vanilla extract
- 10 pitted dates
- a large pinch of Himalayan salt

Directions:

Add all ingredients into blender. Chop mangoes to help with blitzing. You'll definitely enjoy this one. It's a yummy, delicious treat.

Helpful Tips: Add A Powder

Adding powders to your juices works well. Make sure they are reputable brands and are not laced with sugar, salt and/or additives.

Amazing Facts: Himalayan Salt

Himalayan salt is great for health. It acts as an aid in: detoxification, hydration, reducing muscle cramps, balancing blood sugar levels, and balancing systematic PH for cellular health.

Chapter Twenty-Four

RECIPE #24: YUMMY TUMMY

Ingredient List:

- ½ lime, peeled
- 2 apples, any type except Granny Smiths (not great juicers)
- ½ pineapple
- ½ cucumber
- ½ avocado
- Half head of bok choy
- 1 oz. fresh wheatgrass or wheatgrass powder
- 1 level teaspoon of spirulina

Directions:

Juice the apples, pineapple, cucumber, and lime. Put the avocado into juicer. Now add bok choy, wheatgrass and spirulina. Blend everything until smooth, and just pour and enjoy.

Helpful Tips: Blitz with A Friend

Friendship is important, and if you can make your juices with a friend then you'll not only promote health, but you can have fun while you do it! Experiment and laugh as you go!

Amazing Facts: Spirulina is Super-Special

Spirulina is amazing! It has 2800% more beta-carotene than carrots and 3900% more iron than spinach. It's rich in vitamins A, K, K1, K2, B12, and contains manganese and chromium.

Chapter Twenty-Five

RECIPE #25: TANGY COMBO

Ingredient List:

- ½ small pineapple
- ½ stick celery
- 1-inch chunk of cucumber
- 1 small handful of spinach leaves
- 1 peeled lime
- 2 apples
- ½ ripe avocado
- a small handful of parsley

Directions:

Blitz all ingredients until they are smooth and silky. Pour into glass and enjoy.

Helpful Tips: Do It Every Day

Juicing every day is beneficial for long-term health as well as weight loss promotion. Tell your family and friends so they can be healthier too! Juicing is awesome! It's kid-friendly as well.

Amazing Facts: Luscious Limes

Limes are great for health. They have a refined taste and are also jam-packed full of goodness. Great for weight loss promotion, improving digestion, reducing respiratory disorders, constipation relief, and the treatment of: gout, peptic ulcers, scurvy, piles, and gum problems. Whoa! Just amazing!

Chapter Twenty-Six

RECIPE #26: THE PERFECT BLEND

Ingredient List:

- 2 apples
- ½ cucumber
- 1 stick celery
- 1 small handful of spinach
- 1 orange

Directions:

Juice the orange, apples, cucumber, celery and spinach. Add any garnish you wish. Enjoy with or without ice.

Helpful Tips: Work Out First

I like to work out before drinking my juice. Then the healing benefits can take place with the aid of my juice as a healer/energizer. It's great to use juices beforehand, too. It's totally up to you!

Amazing Facts: Summer Workouts

Exercise is great for weight loss. I like to do my workouts in the morning and the evening when the temperature is cooler in the summertime! Add your favorite juice and "Voila!" you can aid health, replenish energy, and lose weight. I love that!

Chapter Twenty-Seven

RECIPE #27: PINEAPPLE PASSION TWISTER

Ingredient List:

- ½ large pineapple
- 2 apples
- ½ cup of alfalfa sprouts
- ½ cup of watercress
- ½ cup of fresh parsley
- ½ cup of kale
- ½ cup of broccoli

Directions:

Blitz all the ingredients. Pour into a glass over ice. Then garnish, serve and enjoy.

Helpful Tips: Add More

I like to add alfalfa and parsley to everything. They both go with most dishes and they're great for juicing as well. Try them as an addition and see if you love them too!

Amazing Facts: Yummy Alfalfa

Alfalfa is beneficial to health. It aids high cholesterol, asthma, osteoarthritis, diabetes, rheumatoid arthritis, and upset stomachs. The benefits are amazing! Mind-blowing really.

Chapter Twenty-Eight

RECIPE #28: YOGURT TROPICANA

Ingredient List:

- ½ small pineapple
- 1 apple
- ½ banana
- 200g natural organic yogurt (soya yogurt)
- ½ teaspoon spirulina

Directions:

Juice the pineapple and apple first. Now add the banana, yogurt and spirulina. Blitz until smooth. Serve and enjoy.

Helpful Tips: Create Your Favorite Juice

Create your favorite juice by adding in ingredients you love. You can try until you get it just right. It's loads of fun and you can give it a great name too!

Amazing Facts: Chamomile Tea

Drinking chamomile tea before meals can aid digestion. Chamomile also has anti-inflammatory and antioxidant qualities. It's also very calming too. A great addition to any diet or health regime.

Chapter Twenty-Nine

RECIPE #29: WARM APPLE-CINNAMON

Ingredient List:

- 3 apples
- 1 good pinch of cinnamon

Directions:

Juice the apples and pour juice into a saucepan. Slowly heat and pour into a mug, then just add cinnamon and serve. Great in the winter.

Helpful Tips: Workouts Inside

If it's cooler weather, you can utilize the inside of your home for workouts. You can dance, do aerobics and stretch too. Go outside if the weather is pleasurable.

Amazing Facts: Wonderful Walking

Walking is great to aid the body in stress relief and weight manage-ment. Walking can also aid insomnia and keep you on track with a healthy heart. Being outside in nature is wonderful!

Chapter Thirty

RECIPE #30: GINGER ZINGER

Ingredient List:

- 2 carrots
- 2 apples
- 1-inch slice of lemon, wax-free, with rind left on
- ½ an inch of fresh ginger

Directions:

Simply juice all ingredients and pour into a glass over ice. Garnish with lemon or celery.

Helpful Tips: Say "Yes" to Yoga

Practicing yoga is great. The health benefits are off the chart for mental, physical and spiritual health. Yoga also calms the body and can aid in healing and longevity too, according to many great studies in recent times.

Amazing Facts: Perfect Apples

Apples are awesome because they come in so many varieties, shapes and sizes. "An apple a day keeps the doctor away!" What a great line. Apples contain loads of vitamins and minerals and can add flavor to juices and meals. They really are so versatile. I love apples!

Chapter Thirty-One

RECIPE #31: GOODNESS GRACIOUS GREENS

Ingredient List:

- 2 sticks of celery
- ½ cucumber
- 1 small handful of spinach
- 1 slice of orange

Directions:

Juice the celery, cucumber and spinach. Add ice to a glass and pour in the pure green super juice. Garnish and suck the orange intermittently, for taste.

Helpful Tips: Add Seeds for More Benefits

Adding chia seeds, sunflower seeds, flaxseed seeds or other types of seeds to your juices is awesome! Packed full of nutrients, seeds can accentuate any juice with their preventative qualities and healing effects.

Amazing Facts: Antioxidants

Antioxidants help to fight molecules and free radicals that move around the body. Foods high in antioxidants help to curb atherosclerosis, cancer, and many other severe conditions.

Chapter Thirty-Two

RECIPE #32: MIND-BLOWING JUICE

Ingredient List:

- 2 apples
- a small piece of carrot
- ½ stick celery
- 1 large handful of mixed green leaves (choose seasonally)
- 1-inch chunk of cucumber
- ½ an inch of broccoli stem
- 1 handful of alfalfa sprouts
- ½ an inch slice of beetroot
- 1 small piece of lemon
- ½ an inch of sliced ginger

Directions:

Juice all the ingredients. Blitz well. Pour over ice and enjoy.

Helpful Tips: Spice Up Your Life

Adding spices to meals can aid in weight loss. Jalapenos are great for that. Make it hotter for more benefit.

Amazing Facts: Healing Broccoli

Broccoli is a wonderful addition to juices and regular meals. Broccoli aids the body in building collagen, and collagen is the substance that forms tissue and bone. Wounds and cuts also need collagen for healing too.

Chapter Thirty-Three

RECIPE #33: GOLDEN DELICIOUS SHERBET

Ingredient List:

- 2 Golden Delicious apples
- 1/3 of a lemon – where possible, wax free and with the rind on

Directions:

Juice the apples and lemon, and pour over ice. Drink and enjoy adding your favorite garnish.

Helpful Tips: Juice for Three Meals with Snacks

Utilize juicing for breakfast, lunch and dinner is awesome. Then add a meat, chicken or fish with the juice. I love doing this. It's super-cool and easy to do, too.

Amazing Facts: Juicing Rocks

Healthy, nutritious, detoxifying, promotes weight loss, and is super fun. Juicing is the healthiest wat to live. I love it! And I know you will too.

Chapter Thirty-Four

RECIPE #34: EFFERVESCENT TASTY

Ingredient List:

- 3 apples
- 1 stick of celery
- half a cucumber
- spinach (1 handful)
- lettuce (1 handful)
- 2 carrots
- ice cubes

Directions:

Peel the apples and the cucumber. Dice them into cubes. Add lettuce and spinach. Add ice and blend it for a minute or so. Drink nice and cold.

Helpful Tips: Keep Knives Sharp

Sounds silly, but there's nothing more frustrating than a blunt knife in the kitchen. Keep them sharp for ease of use and make sure they are kept well-away from children too. Safety first, always.

Amazing Facts: Luscious Lettuce

Lettuce is, quite literally, jam-packed full of great vitamins and minerals. Calcium, iron, magnesium, potassium, sodium, phosphorous, zinc, and vitamins too. So great for you! Add it to everything.

Chapter Thirty-Five

RECIPE #35: LIME AND TANGO

Ingredient List:

- 1/3 of a pineapple
- half a cucumber
- spinach (1 handful)
- 2 apples
- the juice of 2 limes
- ice cubes
- a pinch of Himalayan salt

Directions:

Juice the lime separately in juicer and pour over ice. This helps prevent oxidization of the juice. Chop pineapple and apples and add to the lime ice. Drink and enjoy.

Helpful Tips: Fun with Ice

Have some fun with your ice. Make ice in different shapes by purchasing fun ice trays. Love hearts, bunny rabbits, or even stars look really cool. The kids can have fun too, especially in the summertime.

Amazing Facts: Praising Phosphorous

Phosphorous is great. It aids the body in maintaining: strong bones, detoxification, balancing the PH, energy levels, and is necessary for proper cognitive functioning. Foods high in phosphorous include: salmon, yogurt, nuts, sunflower seeds, and lentils.

Chapter Thirty-Six

RECIPE #36: LOVELY MIXED GREENS

Ingredient List:

- 2 oranges
- 2 carrots
- 1/4 of a lettuce
- 1 celery
- 1/4 of a cabbage
- 2 large branches of broccoli

Directions:

Add carrots, celery, cabbage, and lettuce through the juicer. Stir to blend well with ice, and enjoy. Add any garnishes you require.

Helpful Tips: Help Others Learn

It's never too late to teach others about healthy living. Teach your family, friends and even neighbors so that they can benefit from juicing too. If you want to, you could arrange to talk to kids at a local school so that they can learn about healthy living. You'd need to arrange it first, of course.

Amazing Facts: Vitamin C is Clever

Vitamin C is super-cool. It's necessary for the growth, development and the repair of all body tissues. Vitamin C helps to form collagen, helps absorb iron, and also helps to maintain the cartilage, bones and the teeth. Wow!

Chapter Thirty-Seven

RECIPE #37: KIWI SURPRISE

Ingredient List:

- 2 apples
- 1/3 of a pineapple
- 2 kiwi fruits
- 2 nectarines

Directions:

Remove the stones from the nectarines and the pineapple skin. Chop the pineapple and apples. Add ice, mix well, and drink immediately.

Helpful Tips: Living for Health

When you decide that your health is important your whole world changes. Once you start living to maintain it, you begin to look better, feel better and have more energy.

Amazing Facts: Vitamin K is Colossal

Vitamin K is wonderful. Found in a variety of foods including: kale, spinach, collard greens, Swiss chard, parsley, and green lettuce. It regulates blood clotting and transports calcium throughout the body. It can aid in the decrease of bone fractures and bone density loss.

Chapter Thirty-Eight

RECIPE #38: YUMMY TONIC

Ingredient List:

- 2 carrots
- 1 cucumber
- parsley (1 small bunch)
- spinach (1/2 bunch)
- kale (1 bunch)
- 1 stick of celery
- the juice of a lime
- ice cubes

Directions:

Squeeze the lime first and put on ice cubes. Juice other ingredients and pour over lime and ice. Mix and slowly sip while the ice melts.

Helpful Tips: Keeping Balanced

Most of us have heard about keeping a good work/life balance. It's really important to wind down after work or parenting (a huge job in itself). Meditation, yoga, juicing, and exercise can help to aid health and balance you out.

Amazing Facts: Vitamin A is Astral

Vitamin A is found in a variety of foods. Carrots, sweet potato, kale spinach, broccoli, and eggs too! A great anti-inflammatory and neurological functioning promoter.

Chapter Thirty-Nine

RECIPE #39: MANDARIN MELLOW

Ingredient List:

- 1 orange
- 3 celery sticks
- 1 mandarin

Directions:

Peel orange and mandarin, then chop celery into pieces. Blitz and serve with or without ice. Add a garnish if required.

Helpful Tips: Get Motivated with Music

Getting motivated can be hard sometimes. A great trick I like to use is to listen to music while doing something I don't enjoy. You can put earphones in and listen while doing dishes, exercising, or even cooking.

Amazing Facts: Vitamin B1 is Bountiful

Vitamin B1 is found in green peas, asparagus, brussel sprouts, sesame seeds, sunflower seeds, and crimini mushrooms. Vitamin B1 is vital in maintaining a healthy nervous system, improving cardiovascular functioning, and is necessary for the breakdown of protein and fats in the body.

Chapter Forty

RECIPE #40: ORANGE AND SUBLIME

Ingredient List:

- 2 kiwi fruits
- 1 orange
- 2 apples
- 1 handful of spinach
- 1 carrot
- 1 tablespoon of honey

Directions:

Chop and peel orange and kiwi fruit. Add chopped apples and the spinach with honey. Blitz and serve to enjoy.

Helpful Tips: Use More Honey

I am a bit of a sweet tooth. I like to sweeten everything with honey, and organic is always best, if possible. You can add it to carrots when you cook them, or sweeten your juices with it too. Honey is wonderful.

Amazing Facts: Honey is Whoa-Yeah

Honey is an antibacterial food. It also helps the body to help with weight loss, give energy, promote sleep, heal wounds and ulcers, aid diabetes, and counteracts pollen allergies. What a powerhouse!

Chapter Forty-One

RECIPE #41: YUMMY MONKEY

Ingredient List:

- 3 small apples
- 1 bunch of kale
- 2 carrots
- a pinch of Himalayan salt
- 1 large banana

Directions:

Chop banana, carrot and apples. Add all other ingredients to juicer. Blitz, serve and enjoy. Garnish with lemon or celery as required.

Helpful Tips: Keep Yourself on Target

Write a journal with notes on best recipes, plans, ways to do things, and more. I find that journaling is a great way to combine real life with what you actually do, and with what you want to achieve. And because it's all written down, you can learn or relay back to the information, later on.

Amazing Facts: Niacin is the Best

Niacin helps the body to maintain skin health, support proper brain functioning, improve cholesterol, lower cardiovascular disease risk, and is great to aid joint mobility and to treat arthritis. Niacin is found in: turkey, chicken breast, peanuts, mushrooms, liver, tuna, green peas, and grass-fed beef.

Chapter Forty-Two

RECIPE #42: MANGO MADNESS

Ingredient List:

- 2 mangoes
- 2 apples
- 2 carrots
- 1 handful of alfalfa
- 1 handful of watercress

Directions:

Dice up mangoes, apples and carrots. Place all ingredients into juicer, blitz until silky. Enjoy with or without ice.

Helpful Tips: You Are Worth It

Yes you! I believe in you. And I know you can do this. Whatever you just thought of, just then. Is it weight loss, a new career goal, or something else? I know you can because I did. I lost 100 pounds. Mindset is all you need... keep it positive and motivated. I believe in you!

Amazing Facts: Watercress is Fantastic

Watercress benefits the body in health promotion. It's full of manganese, calcium and antioxidants. A great addition to any meal or juice. I really love this one. Looks amazing too!

Chapter Forty-Three

RECIPE #43: AWESOME FOURSOME

Ingredient List:

- 2 bananas
- 1 mango
- 1 kiwi fruit
- 1 orange
- a handful of parsley

Directions:

Chop all ingredients. Peel kiwi fruit. Add all ingredients to juicer and blitz. You can add a tablespoon of honey to sweeten the taste.

Helpful Tips: Move to Music

You don't need a gym to exercise. Play your favorite album and dance away in your living room... or the bedroom (if you want to keep it between you... and you). Ha! Moving through dance is fun and burns loads of calories too.

Amazing Facts: Mangoes are Magnificent Creations

I love mangoes. They taste great and are great for you. The benefits from mangoes include: lowering cholesterol, clearing skin, alkalizing the entire body, improving digestion, and they also help to fight heat stroke. Cool, huh?

Chapter Forty-Four

RECIPE #44: TANGO ORANGE

Ingredient List:

- 1 orange
- 2 mandarins
- 1 bunch of spinach

Directions:

Peel orange first. Add all of the ingredients to juicer and blitz until soft and silky smooth. Garnish with lemon. Sip and enjoy.

Helpful Tips: Minimize Dairy when Juicing

Loads of calcium comes from fruits and vegetables, and if you want to lose weight, then just minimize or negate dairy. This is especially true to aid in weight loss promotion.

Amazing Facts: Manganese is Amazing

Manganese is needed to help the body form bones and connective tissue. It also aids blood clotting factors and is needed for the sex hormone functioning. Manganese also helps fat and carbohydrate metabolism, and blood sugar regulation.

Chapter Forty-Five

RECIPE #45: CRAZY CARROT JUICE

Ingredient List:

- 6 carrots
- 2 apples
- 1 lemon (with rind)
- a squeeze of lime juice
- 1 tablespoon of honey
- ice cubes

Directions:

Put lime over ice in a glass. Chop apples, carrots and lemon. Add together, then blitz and pour over lime on ice. Enjoy this sweeter with more honey if required.

Helpful Tips: Buy Fresh

If you live close to the grocery store or the market, buy fresh to help minimize waste. It's not fun throwing foods out because they were unused. Fresh and organic is always best.

Amazing Facts: Sweet Potato is Low GI

Although not a major player in juicing, sweet potato is a great low GI food. Instead of using regular potatoes, you can aid your body with this healthier alternative. I love sweet potatoes. They are so versatile. You can boil or roast them, and they give you energy over time. This means they won't be spiking blood sugar levels, which is a big plus.

Chapter Forty-Six

RECIPE #46: GREEN WITH ENVY

Ingredient List:

- 1 handful of kale
- 1 cucumber
- 1 handful of lettuce
- 2 apples
- 1 tablespoon of honey

Directions:

Chop apples and cucumbers into cubes. Add ingredients and blitz. Relax and enjoy with a garnish of your choice.

Helpful Tips: Help a Friend

Once you've got juicing under your wing, you can help others learn the ropes too. Everyone can benefit from the weight loss and healing benefits of juicing. Oh, and detoxification too!

Amazing Facts: Coconut Water is Delightful

Swap out water for coconut water in your juicing recipes. Coconut water is great to help prevent kidney stones, and to support heart health, reduce blood pressure, and it's a big hydrator.

Chapter Forty-Seven

RECIPE #47: THE REAL DEAL

Ingredient List:

- 2 small oranges
- a hint of lemon
- a squeeze of lime juice
- 2 celery sticks

Directions:

Peel oranges first. Chop celery. Blend together and enjoy with or without a garnish, as required.

Helpful Tips: Go All the Way

Yep, keep going until you reach your goal. Whatever it is: weight loss, job promotion, singing karaoke, becoming a parent. You've got this! Yes, you do.

Amazing Facts: Collard Greens

Collard greens are perfect for juicing. They have a high antioxidant quality and they also help the body to stay alkalized. They are loaded with nutrients. Collard greens rock!

Chapter Forty-Eight

RECIPE #48: MANGO MIXER

Ingredient List:

- 3 mangoes
- 2 mandarins
- 2 nectarines
- a squeeze of lemon
- a squeeze of lime

Directions:

Peel and chop mangoes, mandarins and nectarines. Add other ingredients to juicer. Enjoy cold or over ice.

Helpful Tips: Add a Garnish to Make It Fancy

If you want to get a bit fancier, you can add a garnish to your juice. Carrot, celery, tomato, lemon, and orange work well. You can also sprinkle seeds or coconut flakes on top. Yummy!

Amazing Facts: Weight Loss Is Beneficial

When you are at a healthy weight, your body can function at higher levels. The heart load is reduced, and the body feels more energized too. So, make a plan, and get going with it as soon as you can. I have total faith that you can achieve your goal, whatever it might be!

Chapter Forty-Nine

RECIPE #49: APPLE CRAZY

Ingredient List:

- 2 Golden Delicious apples
- 2 carrots
- A slice of lemon
- a squeeze of lime

Directions:

Peel and chop apples and carrots. Add lemon and lime to taste. Blitz well. Garnish with a celery stick or lemon, as required.

Helpful Tips: You Rock!

I think I mentioned this earlier, but I want to reiterate it; just in case no one else told you this lately. Just for taking your health into your own hands, I'm so proud of you. You got this! Go you!

Amazing Facts: Kiwi Fruit is Yummy

Kiwi fruit is super-yummy and is loaded with nutrients to aid in health promotion. A great source of fiber, they contain: vitamin C, vitamin K, vitamin E, potassium, folate, and antioxidants too. Wow, yeah!

Chapter Fifty

RECIPE #50: BANANA-MANGO BENDER

Ingredient List:

- 2 bananas
- 3 mangoes
- 1 apple
- 1 tablespoon of honey

Directions:

Chop up bananas and dice mangoes and apple. Add honey and blitz well. This can be garnished with apple or celery.

Helpful Tips: Refrigeration Is Key

I love keeping my fruit refrigerated. Except for bananas, they don't do so well in the fridge. You can break up bananas and place them separately in a bowl; they last longer that way.

Amazing Facts: Loving Bananas

Bananas contain a high level of magnesium which is essential for great heart health. They also contain potassium which helps to lower blood pressure and decrease the risk of heart disease by a whopping 27%.

IN CONCLUSION

Okay, so one quick word on juicing. I feel better, look better, sleep better, have clearer skin, and I have lost loads and loads of weight. Over 100 pounds in weight, actually. And I taught my entire family how to do it! Except for Aunt Louise, because she is too set in her ways. I'll keep trying her... one day!

I think, for me, I noticed the change in my skin first. I looked in the mirror after two weeks of juicing and my complexion was a whole lot clearer. I thought, *wow, that's a first for me.* Normally, I had little bumps and some acne too. Not heaps, but enough to make me want to put makeup on and cover my skin.

I realized it was actually occurring because of the change in the foods and juices I was now consuming, and due to them being pertinent to my body's homeostasis (balance necessary for proper functioning). And so; that meant that my organs would be affected, in a good way, by the changes I'd made. And, the skin is the biggest organ of the whole body.

So, it makes sense that I would see it there, first. It's still good, even now. Many years later. I just love juicing!

Thank you so much for joining me here to discover the great recipes you can use in your health and weight loss journey. I am thrilled that you can use this book for your health, long-term and ongoing. I really hope you find each and every recipe easy to use and great (taste wise). Remember, you can use your own imagination and add some good fats, and even a touch of honey to sweeten if required.

If you ever find a mixture not silky enough to ingest, you can add a few inches of water (fresh; rain or filtered) to help the recipe taste smoother. Remember, your weight loss and health journey are always your own, and I am so glad I could be a vital part of it. Thank you!

Always remember to look after you first and foremost. And, when you do – your energy levels increase, and in turn, you help your body to maintain optimum functioning, so you can feel amazing! Then, if you've got a boyfriend/girlfriend, or a wife/husband... or kids... or animals... or even a huge career, you'll be able to execute your daily routine easier and with health at the forefront, to keep you going like an Energizer bunny!

I am sending you all of the luck, and my sincerest best wishes to you - now and in the future, on your important journey!

Love and light always, *Emma xx*

P.S. Don't forget, if you haven't already read my title, "How I Lost 100 Pounds! My Personal Weight Loss Strategies for Optimum Happiness," make sure you get your FREE copy today. Inside you'll learn exactly how I lost my weight, and the benefits of knowing the must-do nutrition, and other amazing secrets including myths, water weight, cellulite prevention and removal, the only exercise you really need, the ancient and easy technique to help slim you quickly, how to balance meals, and much, much more! I hope you love it. It's my very special gift to you!

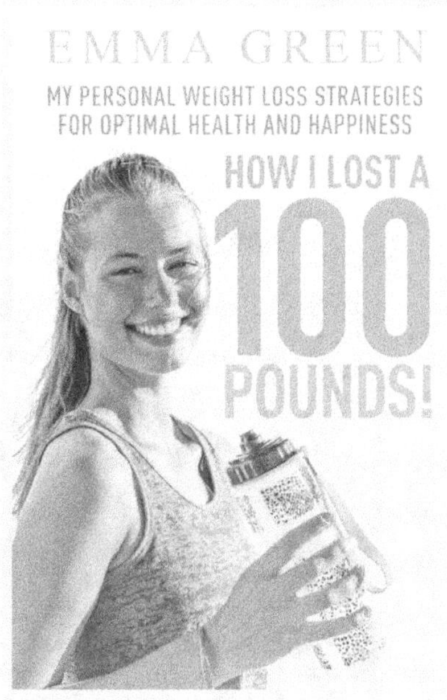

Click here to grab this title absolutely FREE or click on my author profile to checkout my other Free titles.